The Diabetes Reversal for Newly Diagnosed

A Comprehensive Guide to a Life Beyond Type 2

Dr. Billy Norman

Table of Contents

Overview

Diabetes is a persistent condition that arises when the pancreas fails to generate sufficient insulin or when the body is unable to utilize the insulin it produces effectively. Insulin is a hormone responsible for regulating blood glucose levels. Hyperglycemia, characterized by elevated blood glucose or increased blood sugar, is a frequent consequence of unmanaged diabetes. Over time, it can result in severe damage to various systems in the body, particularly the nerves and blood vessels. If you've recently received a diagnosis, or if you're a caregiver seeking solutions for your loved one, this book is your passport to a life beyond the limitations of diabetes. "The Diabetes Reversal Revolution" is more than just a guide; it's a comprehensive roadmap designed to empower and transform.

In this introductory chapter, we embark on a shared quest for understanding, breaking down the walls of confusion and fear that often accompany a diabetes diagnosis. We'll unravel the complexities of type 2 diabetes, exploring not only the science behind it but also the emotional terrain you may navigate. This is the awakening, the moment you reclaim control over your health and embrace the possibility of a future free from the constraints of diabetes.

The first step towards transformation is comprehending the nature of your diagnosis. What does it truly mean to be diagnosed with type 2 diabetes? Beyond the medical terminology, we delve into the emotional impact, recognizing the spectrum of feelings that may arise — from uncertainty and fear to determination and hope.

Building upon this understanding, Chapter 2 takes you on a journey into the heart of type 2 diabetes. Demystifying the condition, we explore the scientific intricacies, providing clarity on how diabetes develops and affects your body. By demystifying blood sugar and its role, we equip you with the knowledge needed to make informed decisions about your health.

As we progress through the chapters, a blueprint for reversal emerges. From lifestyle strategies that form the core of your transformation to overcoming challenges and celebrating successes, each chapter builds upon the last, creating a comprehensive guide to reclaiming your health.

This book is not just a manual; it's an invitation to join the Diabetes Reversal Revolution. Let's break free from the chains of diabetes, embrace a healthier lifestyle, and move confidently towards a non-diabetic future. The journey starts now – are you ready?

Chapter 1

The Basics

In the health field, a fundamental understanding of type 2 diabetes is paramount. Diabetes mellitus, commonly known as diabetes, is a chronic metabolic disorder characterized by elevated blood glucose levels. Type 2 diabetes, in particular, arises when the body becomes resistant to the effects of insulin, a hormone essential for regulating blood sugar. Unlike type 1 diabetes, where the body doesn't produce insulin, type 2 diabetes involves a combination of insulin resistance and relative insulin deficiency.

Types of Diabetes

Prediabetes

In the United States, 84.1 million adults exhibit blood sugar levels higher than normal, falling into the category of prediabetes or impaired glucose tolerance. Prediabetes typically manifests without noticeable symptoms, but it precedes the development of type 2 diabetes. Despite the absence of clear symptoms, complications associated with diabetes, such as heart disease, can commence even during the prediabetes stage. Consult with your doctor to determine if testing for prediabetes is necessary, as proactive measures can potentially prevent the onset of type 2 diabetes and reduce the risk of associated complications like heart disease.

Type 1 Diabetes

Type 1 diabetes results from the immune system attacking and destroying the insulin-producing cells (beta cells) in the pancreas. Individuals with type 1 diabetes do not produce insulin and must rely on insulin injections to regulate their blood sugar levels. While type 1 diabetes commonly emerges in individuals under 20 years of age, it can occur at any age.

Type 2 Diabetes

In contrast to type 1 diabetes, individuals with type 2 diabetes produce insulin. However, either the amount of insulin produced by the pancreas is insufficient, or the body develops insulin resistance. When there is an inadequate supply of insulin or it is not effectively utilized, glucose cannot enter the body's cells. Type 2 diabetes, the most prevalent form, affects nearly 18 million Americans. While preventable in most cases, it remains the leading cause of diabetes-related complications in adults, including blindness, non-traumatic amputations, and chronic kidney failure necessitating dialysis. Although type 2 diabetes typically occurs in individuals over 40 who are overweight, it can also affect those who are not overweight. Often termed "adult-onset diabetes," it has become more prevalent in children due to the rise in childhood obesity. Management of type 2 diabetes may involve weight control, dietary adjustments, regular exercise, and, in some cases, medication or insulin injections. Detecting the likelihood of type 2 diabetes before its onset, commonly referred to as pre-diabetes, involves identifying elevated blood sugar levels that are not yet diagnostic for type 2 diabetes.

Gestational Diabetes

Gestational diabetes arises during pregnancy, influenced by hormonal changes that impact insulin function. Approximately 9% of all pregnancies experience this condition. Pregnant women at an elevated risk of developing gestational diabetes include those over 25 years old, with a pre-pregnancy body weight above normal, a family history of diabetes, or belonging to ethnic groups such as Hispanic, black, Native American, or Asian. Screening for gestational diabetes is conducted during pregnancy to mitigate potential complications for both the mother and the unborn child. Although blood sugar levels typically normalize within six weeks after childbirth, women with a history of gestational diabetes face an increased risk of developing type 2 diabetes later in life.

To comprehend type 2 diabetes fully, it's essential to explore the intricate dance between insulin, glucose, and the body's cells. Insulin acts as the key, unlocking cells to allow glucose entry for energy production. In type 2 diabetes, this process becomes impaired, leading to an accumulation of glucose in the bloodstream.

Causes and Risk Factors

1. Genetic Predisposition

While genetics play a role in diabetes susceptibility, having a family history of the condition doesn't guarantee its development. Understanding genetic predisposition empowers individuals to make informed lifestyle choices for diabetes prevention.

2. Lifestyle Factors and Obesity

Lifestyle choices significantly contribute to the development of type 2 diabetes. Poor dietary habits, sedentary lifestyles, and obesity are major culprits. Excess weight, particularly around the abdomen, is associated with insulin resistance, a precursor to type 2 diabetes.

3. Metabolic Syndrome and Insulin Resistance

Metabolic syndrome, a cluster of conditions including elevated blood pressure, high blood sugar, excess body fat, and abnormal cholesterol levels, often precedes type 2 diabetes. Insulin resistance, where cells don't respond effectively to insulin, is a central component.

Common Symptoms of Type 2 Diabetes

Recognizing the symptoms is pivotal for early diagnosis. These may include increased thirst, frequent urination, unexplained weight loss, fatigue, Numbness in the feet, excessive hunger and blurred vision. Awareness of these signs prompts timely medical evaluation.

Diagnostic Tests and Blood Sugar Levels

Diagnostic tests, including fasting blood sugar and oral glucose tolerance tests, help confirm a diabetes diagnosis. Monitoring blood sugar levels provides insights into the severity of the condition and guides treatment strategies.

Importance of Early Detection

Early detection enables prompt intervention, reducing the risk of complications. Timely lifestyle modifications and, if necessary, medical interventions can significantly impact the trajectory of the disease.

Chapter 2

Understanding Your Diagnosis

In the quiet corridors of a diagnosis room, life takes an unexpected turn. A diagnosis of type 2 diabetes is more than a medical verdict; it's an invitation to a journey of self-discovery and empowerment. This chapter serves as the threshold to this transformative expedition, guiding you through the labyrinth of medical intricacies and emotional landscapes that accompany a diabetes diagnosis.

The diagnosis of type 2 diabetes introduces you to a new lexicon of medical terminology and physiological intricacies.

The human body operates like a finely tuned orchestra, with various systems harmoniously working together. However, when the conductor, in this case, insulin, faces resistance, the melody of balance falters, and type 2 diabetes takes center stage.

We unravel this clinical tapestry, exploring the dynamics of blood sugar regulation, insulin production, and the interplay of genetics and lifestyle factors in the development of diabetes.

Through relatable examples and clear explanations, we bridge the gap between medical concepts and everyday understanding. Imagine insulin as the key unlocking the door to your body's cells, allowing glucose to enter and provide energy. In diabetes, this process encounters obstacles, leading to elevated blood sugar levels. As we navigate this metaphorical journey, you gain insights into the factors influencing insulin resistance and the delicate balance required for metabolic harmony.

Understanding your diagnosis involves interpreting the clues embedded in diagnostic tests. We demystify the significance of blood glucose levels, HbA1c, and lipid profiles, providing you with a roadmap to comprehend your health markers. By gaining insight into these test results, you not only grasp the current state of your health but also lay the groundwork for proactive decision-making.

From fasting blood sugar tests to oral glucose tolerance tests, we navigate the various diagnostic tools used by healthcare professionals. You'll learn how these tests unveil the story of your metabolic health and why each piece of information is crucial in guiding your personalized care plan. Armed with this knowledge, you become an active participant in your healthcare journey, equipped to ask informed questions and collaborate with your healthcare team.

Beyond the clinical parameters and medical charts, a type 2 diabetes diagnosis triggers a profound emotional journey. In this section, we delve into the intricate landscape of feelings and psychological responses that accompany the news of a diabetes diagnosis, acknowledging that emotional well-being is an integral part of your overall health.

Receiving a diagnosis is akin to stepping onto a rollercoaster of emotions, each twist and turn bringing forth a range of feelings. From the initial shock and disbelief to the subtle currents of anxiety and fear, we recognize the emotional terrain that is often traversed in the wake of a diabetes diagnosis. It's essential to acknowledge these emotions without judgment, understanding that they are valid responses to a significant life event.

Through shared narratives and personal stories, we connect on a human level. Others have walked this path before you, facing similar emotional challenges. By hearing their stories, you gain insights into the emotional journey, discovering that you are not alone in your experience. These stories are not just accounts of struggle but testaments to resilience and the capacity of the human spirit to adapt and overcome.

Within the emotional landscape, we explore coping mechanisms that can serve as beacons of light during challenging times. Whether it's through mindfulness practices, creative outlets, or simply finding solace in the support of loved ones, you'll discover a diverse toolkit to navigate the emotional journey. By fostering self-awareness and emotional intelligence, you empower yourself to respond to the diagnosis with resilience and grace.

Additionally, we delve into real-world examples of individuals who have embraced their emotional journey, sharing how they navigated the complex terrain of emotions associated with a diabetes diagnosis. These narratives provide not only inspiration but also practical insights into how emotional challenges can be transformed into opportunities for growth and self-discovery.

Chapter 3

How to Reverse Type 2 Diabetes

Type 2 diabetes currently lacks a definitive cure, though research indicates that certain individuals can effectively reverse its effects. This reversal is often achieved through significant modifications to one's diet and weight loss, potentially enabling the maintenance of normal blood sugar levels without the need for medication.

It is crucial to note that while achieving remission by managing diet and weight can be impactful, it doesn't signify complete eradication of the condition. Type 2 diabetes is a persistent ailment, and even during remission, there exists a possibility of symptoms resurfacing. Nevertheless, some individuals successfully control their glucose levels for extended periods, experiencing years without the complications associated with diabetes.

The key element in reversing diabetes appears to be weight loss. Shedding excess pounds not only aids in diabetes management but, in some cases, could lead to a diabetes-free state, particularly for individuals diagnosed within the last few years and not requiring insulin.

Research on the effects of a very low-calorie diet demonstrated promising outcomes for overweight individuals with diabetes. Participants followed a predominantly liquid diet of 625-850 calories per day for 2-5 months, followed by a less restrictive diet to help them maintain their weight loss. Nearly half of the participants in these studies successfully reversed their diabetes, sustaining normal blood glucose levels for a significant period.

It's important to acknowledge that such an extreme diet necessitates professional guidance and meticulous calorie control. While challenging, the potential for diabetes remission serves as a compelling motivation to adhere to this approach.

Most individuals who achieved diabetes reversal through weight loss lost 30 pounds or more and had a shorter history of diabetes. Therefore, early initiation of a weight loss plan is recommended for those newly diagnosed.

In individuals with type 2 diabetes, the malfunctioning of cells that regulate blood sugar is a primary concern. Weight loss, particularly a reduction in liver and pancreas fat levels, may contribute to the reactivation of beta cells in the pancreas responsible for insulin release. The likelihood of reviving these cells is highest during the early stages of diabetes, emphasizing the importance of substantial weight loss post-diagnosis rather than relying solely on lifestyle changes and medication.

Exercise plays a significant role in improving diabetes outcomes. While increasing physical activity alone may not be sufficient to achieve remission, when combined with dietary modifications, exercise becomes a valuable component. A study incorporating a goal of 10,000 steps a day, at least 3 hours of moderate exercise weekly, a 500-750 calorie reduction per day, and adherence to a specific insulin and medication routine showed over half of the participants reaching near-normal blood sugar levels without medication. This underscores the importance of weight loss, with exercise serving as a complementary factor in achieving diabetes remission.

Chapter 4

Lifestyle Change for Diabetes Reversal

In the modern era, where sedentary lifestyles and processed foods have become the norm, the prevalence of diabetes has reached alarming levels. However, hope shines through the shadows, as emerging research highlights the potential for diabetes reversal through a holistic lifestyle change. This comprehensive guide explores the multifaceted approach to transforming your life and reversing diabetes through mindful choices in diet, physical activity, stress management, and sleep hygiene.

Dietary Modifications

The foundation of any lifestyle change for diabetes reversal lies in adopting a balanced and nutrient-dense diet. Focus on incorporating whole, unprocessed foods such as fruits, vegetables, whole grains, and lean proteins into your daily meals. Emphasize foods with a low glycemic index to help stabilize blood sugar levels. Limit your intake of refined sugars, saturated fats, and processed foods, as they can contribute to insulin resistance.

Consider adopting a Mediterranean or plant-based diet, which has been shown to have profound effects on improving insulin sensitivity. These diets are rich in antioxidants, fiber, and healthy fats, which collectively support better blood sugar control and overall metabolic health.

In addition to embracing a balanced diet, consider incorporating specific foods known for their diabetes-fighting properties. Foods rich in omega-3 fatty acids, such as fatty fish (salmon, mackerel), chia seeds, and flaxseeds, have been shown to improve insulin sensitivity. Nuts, especially almonds and walnuts, are excellent snacks that provide healthy fats, fiber, and essential nutrients.

Experiment with herbs and spices like cinnamon, turmeric, and ginger, which have anti-inflammatory properties and may contribute to better blood sugar control. Green tea, with its antioxidants, can also be a refreshing beverage choice that aligns with your diabetes reversal goals.

Hydration is often overlooked but plays a crucial role in overall health. Opt for water as your primary beverage, and limit sugary drinks and excessive caffeine intake. Proper hydration supports kidney function, helps regulate blood sugar levels, and aids in weight management.

Importance of Diet

a. **Balanced Nutrition**

Achieving diabetes reversal hinges significantly on adopting a diet that prioritizes balanced nutrition. Understanding the role of macronutrients—carbohydrates, proteins, and fats—is essential for making informed dietary choices.

- **Carbohydrates:** Recognize the impact of different carbohydrates on blood sugar levels. Opt for complex carbohydrates found in whole grains, fruits, and vegetables, which release glucose more slowly, helping to maintain stable blood sugar.

- **Proteins:** Include lean protein sources such as poultry, fish, beans, and tofu. Protein not only supports muscle health but also helps in managing hunger and stabilizing blood sugar.

- **Fats:** Emphasize healthy fats like those found in avocados, nuts, and olive oil. These fats contribute to overall well-being and help regulate insulin sensitivity.

- **Fiber:** Prioritize fiber-rich foods, including whole grains, legumes, fruits, and vegetables. Fiber aids in digestion, helps control blood sugar levels, and promotes a feeling of fullness.

b. Portion Control

Effective diabetes management involves not just what you eat but also how much. Portion control is crucial for preventing overconsumption, stabilizing blood sugar levels, and managing weight.

- **Understanding Portion Sizes:** Educate yourself on recommended portion sizes for different food groups. This awareness assists in preventing unintentional overeating and contributes to better blood sugar control.

- **Tools for Portion Control:** Utilize tools such as measuring cups, a food scale, or visual cues to estimate portion sizes accurately. These aids empower you to maintain control over your food intake.

- **Identifying Overeating Triggers:** Recognize emotional and environmental triggers that may lead to overeating. Developing strategies to cope with these triggers is pivotal in cultivating a healthier relationship with food.

c. Meal Planning

Crafting a well-thought-out meal plan is a cornerstone of diabetes reversal. A structured approach to meals helps manage blood sugar levels effectively.

- **Glycemic Index Awareness:** Consider the glycemic index of foods, which indicates how quickly they raise blood sugar. Favor low to moderate glycemic index foods to avoid sharp spikes in blood glucose.

- **Timing of Meals:** Establish a consistent meal schedule. Spacing meals evenly throughout the day can prevent drastic fluctuations in blood sugar levels and provide sustained energy.

- **Variety for Optimal Nutrition:** Introduce a variety of foods to ensure a broad spectrum of nutrients. This not only supports overall health but also contributes to sustained dietary adherence.

Regular Physical Activity

Engaging in regular physical activity is a cornerstone of diabetes reversal. Aim for at least 150 minutes of moderate-intensity aerobic exercise per week, along with strength training exercises two to three times per week. Exercise helps your body utilize glucose more efficiently, improves insulin sensitivity, and contributes to weight management.

Find activities you enjoy, whether it's brisk walking, cycling, swimming, or dancing. Incorporate movement into your daily routine, such as taking the stairs instead of the elevator or going for a short walk after meals to aid digestion and regulate blood sugar levels.

Stress Management

Chronic stress can negatively impact blood sugar levels and exacerbate diabetes. Implement stress-reducing techniques such as meditation, deep breathing exercises, yoga, or tai chi into your daily routine. These practices not only help lower stress hormones but also improve overall mental well-being.

Establishing a healthy work-life balance and setting realistic goals can contribute to stress reduction. Prioritize self-care activities that bring joy and relaxation, such as spending time in nature, reading, or pursuing hobbies.

Adequate Sleep

Quality sleep is essential for diabetes reversal. Aim for 7-9 hours of uninterrupted sleep each night. Poor sleep can disrupt hormonal balance, leading to insulin resistance and increased cravings for unhealthy foods. Create a conducive sleep environment by keeping the bedroom dark, cool, and quiet, and establish a consistent sleep schedule.

Avoid stimulants like caffeine and electronic devices before bedtime, as they can interfere with sleep quality. If sleep problems persist, consult a healthcare professional for guidance.

Regular Monitoring and Medical Check-ups

Regular monitoring of blood sugar levels is crucial for tracking progress and making necessary adjustments to your lifestyle change plan. Work closely with your healthcare team to develop an individualized approach, and attend regular check-ups to assess your overall health and diabetes management.

Mindful Eating

Practicing mindful eating can be a powerful tool in your diabetes reversal journey. Slow down during meals, savor each bite, and pay attention to hunger and fullness cues. This approach helps prevent overeating, encourages healthier food choices, and promotes a positive relationship with food. Consider keeping a food journal to track your meals, snacks, and emotional triggers related to eating. This can provide valuable insights into your dietary habits and help you make informed choices for sustainable lifestyle changes.

Community Support

Embarking on a lifestyle change for diabetes reversal can be challenging, but you don't have to face it alone. Seek support from friends, family, or join community groups or online forums where individuals share their experiences and tips. Connecting with others on a similar journey can provide motivation, encouragement, and a sense of camaraderie.

Educate yourself about diabetes through reputable sources and stay informed about the latest research and lifestyle strategies. Attend workshops or support groups to enhance your knowledge and receive guidance from healthcare professionals specializing in diabetes management.

Celebrate Achievements

Recognize and celebrate your achievements along the way, whether they involve improved blood sugar levels, weight loss, increased energy, or better overall well-being. Setting realistic, short-term goals can provide a sense of accomplishment and keep you motivated throughout your diabetes reversal journey.

Remember that the path to diabetes reversal is unique for each individual. Be patient with yourself, stay committed to your lifestyle changes, and celebrate the progress you make. With dedication and a holistic approach, you have the power to not only manage but potentially reverse diabetes, reclaiming a healthier and more vibrant life.

Chapter 5

Monitoring blood sugar level

Monitoring blood sugar levels is a critical aspect of managing type 2 diabetes. Regular and accurate monitoring empowers individuals to make informed decisions about their lifestyle, diet, and medication adjustments. Blood sugar monitoring is a dynamic process, and the insights gained from consistent tracking play a crucial role in effectively managing type 2 diabetes. Regular communication with your healthcare team and proactive adjustments to your lifestyle based on these insights are key components of successful diabetes management.

Here's a short guide on monitoring blood sugar levels for type 2 diabetes:

1. **Frequency of Monitoring:**

   - **Daily Monitoring:** Check your blood sugar levels regularly as advised by your healthcare provider. Typically, this involves testing before meals and possibly after meals, as well as at other specific times during the day.

- **A1c Test:** This test, usually done every three to six months, provides an average of your blood sugar levels over an extended period. It offers a more comprehensive view of your overall diabetes management.

2. **Choosing a Glucometer:**

- Select a reliable glucometer that suits your needs and is easy to use. Ensure it is properly calibrated and consult with your healthcare team for recommendations.

- Modern glucometers often come with features like memory storage, which allows you to track trends in your blood sugar levels over time.

3. **Testing Technique:**

- Wash your hands thoroughly before testing to avoid contamination that may affect the accuracy of the reading.

- Use a lancet to prick the side of your fingertip for a small blood sample. Some individuals prefer alternative testing sites, like the forearm, but always consult with your healthcare provider first.

- Apply the blood sample to the test strip and insert it into the glucometer. Wait for the results, and record them in a logbook or a digital app.

4. **Interpreting Blood Sugar Levels:**

- **Fasting Blood Sugar:** Typically measured in the morning before eating. Normal levels are usually between 70 and 130 mg/dL.

- **Postprandial Blood Sugar:** Measured 1-2 hours after meals. Target levels are generally less than 180 mg/dL.

- **A1c Levels:** The target A1c level is often less than 7%. However, individual targets may vary, and your healthcare provider will guide you based on your specific health status.

5. **Detecting Patterns and Trends:**

- Regular monitoring helps identify patterns and trends in blood sugar levels. This information is valuable for adjusting medication, making dietary modifications, and optimizing lifestyle choices.

- If you notice consistently high or low readings, discuss them with your healthcare team. They can help determine if adjustments to your treatment plan are necessary.

6. **Integration with Lifestyle Changes:**

- Use blood sugar readings to assess the impact of diet, exercise, stress, and medication on your glucose levels.

- Tailor your meal plans and physical activity based on how your body responds to different factors, ensuring a more personalized and effective diabetes management strategy.

7. **Communication with Healthcare Team:**

- Share your blood sugar logs, concerns, and questions with your healthcare provider regularly. This collaboration is essential for making informed decisions about your diabetes management plan.

Chapter 6

Support and Education for Newly Diagnosed

Being diagnosed with diabetes can be a life-altering experience, but with the right support and education, individuals can empower themselves to manage their condition effectively and lead fulfilling lives.

Embarking on the path of managing diabetes as a newly diagnosed individual may seem overwhelming, but with the right support and education, it becomes a journey of empowerment and resilience.

Remember, you are not alone, and there is a wealth of resources and a community ready to help you navigate the challenges and triumphs that lie ahead. Embrace the opportunity to learn, adapt, and lead a fulfilling life with diabetes.

Here are some tips

1. **Professional Guidance:**

- Seek guidance from healthcare professionals, including endocrinologists, diabetes educators, and registered dietitians. These experts can provide essential information about diabetes, explain treatment options, and assist in creating a personalized management plan.

2. **Patient Education Programs:**

- Participate in patient education programs offered by healthcare facilities or community organizations. These programs cover a wide range of topics, including understanding blood sugar levels, medication management, healthy eating, and the importance of regular physical activity.

3. **Online Resources:**

- Explore reputable online resources provided by diabetes associations, medical institutions, and health websites. These platforms offer a wealth of information, from basics about diabetes to tips for daily management, recipes, and success stories from individuals who have effectively managed their condition.

4. **Support Groups:**

- Join diabetes support groups, either in person or online, to connect with others facing similar challenges. Sharing experiences and insights with individuals who understand the emotional and physical aspects of living with diabetes can provide a sense of camaraderie and support.

5. **Family and Friends:**

- Educate your close circle of family and friends about diabetes to foster a supportive environment. Help them understand the challenges you may face and how they can actively contribute to your well-being. Encourage open communication and create a network of allies on your journey.

6. **Psychosocial Support:**

- Recognize the emotional impact of a diabetes diagnosis and consider seeking psychosocial support. Mental health professionals can provide guidance on coping with the emotional aspects of managing a chronic condition, addressing stress, anxiety, and potential feelings of isolation.

7. **Lifestyle Modification Programs:**

- Enroll in lifestyle modification programs that focus on diet, exercise, and stress management. These programs often provide practical tools and strategies for incorporating healthy habits into daily life, promoting overall well-being alongside diabetes management.

8. **Continuous Learning:**

- Diabetes is a dynamic condition, and ongoing education is crucial. Stay informed about new research, treatment options, and lifestyle strategies. Regularly consult with healthcare professionals to adjust your management plan based on evolving needs.

9. **Monitoring and Self-Care Skills:**

- Learn to monitor blood sugar levels and acquire essential self-care skills. Understanding how lifestyle choices impact blood sugar and being proficient in medication management are fundamental aspects of successful diabetes management.

10. Goal Setting and Celebrating Progress:

- Set realistic and achievable goals for your diabetes management. Celebrate small victories, whether they relate to blood sugar control, lifestyle changes, or emotional well-being. Positive reinforcement can be a powerful motivator on your journey.

Conclusion

As we close the pages of this guide for those newly diagnosed with Type 2 Diabetes, remember that this is not the end—it's the beginning of a transformative journey towards a healthier and more empowered you. Armed with knowledge, resilience, and practical strategies, you now possess the tools to reverse the course of diabetes and reclaim control over your health.

Embrace the journey with the mindset that every small change is a victory. From understanding the importance of nutrition to incorporating regular exercise, these steps, no matter how modest, collectively pave the way to a life less dictated by diabetes.

As you move forward, remember that you are not alone. This journey is a shared experience, and there is a community of support around you. Keep learning, stay resilient, and celebrate every milestone, for each one is a step closer to a life free from the constraints of Type 2 Diabetes.

Your story is still being written, and this is just the beginning of a new chapter—one where you take charge of your health, rewrite the narrative, and embrace a future filled with vitality and well-being. Here's to your journey towards a healthier, diabetes-free life.